Dental Erosion

Quintessentials of Dental Practice – 34
Clinical Practice – 4

Dental Erosion

By
R Graham Chadwick

Editor-in-Chief: Nairn H F Wilson
Editor Clinical Practice: Nairn H F Wilson

Quintessence Publishing Co. Ltd.
London, Berlin, Chicago, Paris, Milan, Barcelona, Istanbul,
São Paulo, Tokyo, New Delhi, Moscow, Prague, Warsaw

British Library Cataloguing-in Publication Data

Chadwick, R. Graham
  Dental erosion. – (Quintessentials of dental practice; 34. Clinical practice; 4)
  1. Teeth – Erosion
  I. Title
  617.6´3

ISBN 185097165X

ISBN 1-85097-165-X

Foreword

Dental erosion is increasingly common. The effect of erosion, in particular if generalised, can be profound, with lifelong consequences for the prognosis of the dentition. Given new understanding and knowledge of the aetiology of dental erosion and its management, *Dental Erosion* is a timely and valuable addition to the popular *Quintessentials of Dental Practice* series.

In common with the other carefully targeted books in the series, a modern, evidence-based, preventative approach, underpinned by systematic history taking and diagnosis, is strongly advocated. Mindful of the busy practitioner's time and opportunity to read and digest dental publications, *Dental Erosion* presents the essence of the subject in a concise, well-illustrated, easy-to-read style, highlighting key issues of immediate practical relevance.

With many more patients, notably adolescents and young adults presenting with dental erosion, *Dental Erosion* will be of assistance to practitioners of all ages and levels of experience, seeking to provide their patients with state-of-the-art care. If you are uncertain about aspects of dental erosion observed in your patients, this book will be an excellent addition to your reference texts – another jewel in the *Quintessentials* series crown.

Nairn Wilson
Editor-in-Chief

Acknowledgements

The author would like to acknowledge with sincere thanks the following people and organisations: Mrs Rene Burnett (Dundee Dental School and Hospital) for her photographic skills; Mrs Frances Anderson (Dundee Dental School) for typing the early drafts of the manuscript; Mr Steve Bonsor for proof-reading; Miss Lynne Allan for ensuring the smooth running of my consultant clinics; the dental technicians of Dundee Dental Hospital Conservation Laboratory (Mr Dave McMahon, Mr John McLeish, Mr Donald Aitkenhead, Mr Brian Devine, Mr Kevin Linklater, Mrs Joyce Thomson); Mr Bill Sharp (senior dental instructor, Dundee Dental School), Dr John Radford (Dundee Dental School) for Fig 4-17; Dr Alex Milosevic (Liverpool Dental Hospital) and the editor of the British Dental Journal for Fig 2-2; Professor Jeremy Rees (Cardiff Dental School) for the data in Table 2-2 together with the editor of the European Journal of Prosthodontics and Restorative Dentistry; Dr Andrew Mason (Dundee Dental School) for Fig 4-9; Professor Andrew Grieve for Figs 1-2, 1-3 and 3-1; Dr Julie Kilgariff for her data on attitudes and beliefs surrounding dental erosion; Professor Sue Higham and Gleb Komarov (Liverpool Dental School) for Fig 5-2; the editors of The European Journal of Dental Science (for Tables 2-1, 3-1, 3-2), The Journal of the American Medical Association (for Table 3-5), The British Medical Journal (for Table 3-4) and the press office of www.weight-lossresources.co.uk for the basis of Figs 3-6 and 3-7; the editor of Quintessence International for permission to reproduce Fig 5-3. Also Dr Harvey Mitchell (University of Newcastle, Australia) for his longstanding research collaboration, Tenovus Tayside for funding the research whose data is in Table 3-3, Dr Nick Halpin (Counselling Service, University of Dundee) for his insight into student culture, Mr James Beaton (librarian of the Royal College of Physicians and Surgeons of Glasgow) for facilitating access to texts covering the historical aspects of erosion and both Professor Nairn Wilson (commissioning editor) and the Quintessentials production team for their assistance. Last, but not least, Sandra, Matthew, Benjamin and Nathan for their patience and support.

Contents

'Our information regarding erosion is far from complete, and it now seems probable that much time may elapse before its investigation will have satisfactory results. Its increasing frequency and the great damage it is doing calls for the closest study that the profession can give.'

G. V. Black (1908)

Chapter 1
Erosion – Is it a Problem?

'There are no new truths, but only truths that have not been recognised by those who have perceived them without noticing.'

Mary MacArthur from On The Contrary (1961)

Aim

To appreciate other forms of tooth surface loss, the nature and prevalence of dental erosion.

Outcome

After reading this chapter the reader should have an understanding of:
- other forms of tooth surface loss
- the historical background surrounding dental erosion
- the prevalence of dental erosion
- the limitations of the present evidence base.

Introduction and Historical Background

In its true sense dental erosion may be defined as the loss of enamel and dentine from chemical attack other than those chemicals produced intraorally by bacteria. This distinguishes it from dental caries, in which the damaging acid is produced from the fermentation of carbohydrates and the microorganisms of dental plaque. Although many would attribute the classical appearance of palatal tooth surface loss (Fig 1-1) to this process, it should never be forgotten that such surfaces may also wear due to both abrasion and attrition working in combination with the erosive process. Abrasion is physical wear brought about by contact with objects other than a tooth (Fig 1-2). Attrition is the physical wear of one tooth surface against another, with tooth tissue loss occurring on the contacting surfaces (Fig 1-3). In any patient all three mechanisms may be at work to a lesser or greater extent. As a result the dentist should always conduct a detailed examination to determine the major cause of the tooth surface loss that presents.

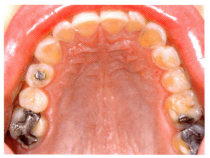

Fig 1-1 Dental erosion affecting the palatal aspects of the maxillary teeth – note also the submargination of the amalgam restorations in UR4, UR6 and UL6.

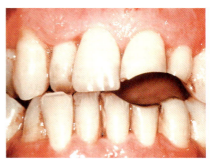

Fig 1-2 Abrasion of the upper and lower incisors produced from contact with a pipe stem over many years.

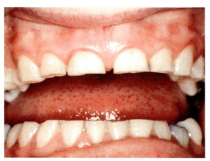

Fig 1-3 Attrition of the dentition of a female patient aged 25 years.

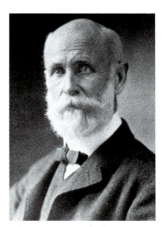

Fig 1-4 G.V. Black.

It is tempting and convenient to believe that dental erosion is a relatively new phenomenon that is the product of modern times. This is untrue - the condition, as defined today, was familiar to dentists at the turn of the 19th century. These included G. V. Black (Fig 1-4). He reported upon the condition in his 1908 work on operative dentistry. This makes remarkable reading, because he states that 'erosion is rarer than dental caries but more frequent in the more affluent classes'. He also suggested that once practitioners were familiar with dental erosion they would see more cases. Rather farsightedly he postulated that the individual susceptibility to the condition he witnessed may have a hereditary basis. He commented that although erosion tended to progress slowly this could cease spontaneously or continue intermittently. These observations were pertinent, holding true today. They pose a number of dilemmas for today's practitioner. Should all patients be given the same preventive advice? When should erosion be operatively treated or the impact of preventive measures observed?

Typically dental erosion manifests itself in late adolescence or early adulthood. This is at a time when patients tend to be acutely concerned about their life style and appearance. They also have many years of life ahead of them. As a result the management of such patients presents a considerable challenge to the dentist. When today's restoration is placed it will ultimately fail at some stage in the future. Will the mode of failure facilitate or hinder recovery? Clinical management options selected now must keep future treatment options open. This book seeks to provide a framework of knowledge to enable the dental team to manage this group of patients. It should be regarded as a pick 'n' mix tool box to address such dilemmas for the benefit of individual patients. It is not a prescriptive recipe book of solutions.

Prevalence

Surprisingly, few studies have examined the prevalence of dental erosion. Although it is generally accepted that the prevalence is highest in young people and adolescents, it is not always possible to compare the findings of one study with another. This is due to the different methods of recording erosion used by each group of researchers. It is therefore difficult to get a picture of the problem. The most comprehensive epidemiological data originates from the UK.

The 1993 National Survey of UK Child Dental Health reported that nearly 25% of 11-year-olds and 50% of five- to six-year-olds exhibited dental erosion. Similar proportions of young people, aged four to 18 years, were found to have dental erosion in the UK National Diet and Nutrition Surveys published in 2000. Interestingly this study also found no consistent relationship between the frequency of intake of either sugary or acid foods and dental erosion. They also commented that those who consume drinks quickly were as likely to have erosion as those who made drinks last over a prolonged period. This flies in the face of our present-day understanding of the condition where frequent intakes of acid are thought to prolong the duration of the acidic challenge, thereby increasing the erosion risk. This highlights the need for further research to improve our understanding of the condition.

Clearly, if the erosive process continues throughout adulthood there is a major problem, as considerable amounts of tooth substance will be lost.

The recent UK 2003 Children's Dental Health Survey reported a slight increase in the proportion (14%) of 15-year-olds exhibiting erosive tooth surface loss on the buccal aspects of the incisors. There was, however, a 6% increase, since that reported in the 1993 Survey, in the proportion (33%) of individuals with the lingual aspect of the teeth affected by erosion. As in 1993, however, very few involved dentine or pulp. Of those surveyed 22% demonstrated occlusal erosion of the first molars, with 4% involving dentine.

Outwith the UK, some 7.7% of Swiss adults (aged 26–30 years) have been reported as having at least one tooth with buccal erosion. Some 3.6% have slight lingual erosion of the maxillary anterior teeth. Although severe lingual erosion is said to be scarce, some 2.9% display at least one site of severe occlusal erosion.

A recent survey that compared the prevalence of erosion affecting the upper permanent incisors, in 11–13-year-olds, in the UK and the USA suggested a similar prevalence for both countries (UK, 37%; USA, 41%).

Further Reading

Chadwick B, Pendry L. Non-Carious Dental Conditions – Children's Dental Health in the United Kingdom, 2003. London: Office for National Statistics, 2004.

Deery C, Wagner M L, Longbottom C et al. The prevalence of dental erosion in a United States and a United Kingdom sample of adolescents. Pediatr Dent 2000;22:505-510.

Lussi A, Schaffner M, Hotz P, Suter P Dental Erosion in a population of Swiss adults. Community Dent Oral Epidemiol 1991;19:286-290.

Nunn J H, Gordon P H, Morris A J et al. Dental erosion – changing prevalence? A review of British National Child Dental Health Surveys. International Journal of Paediatric Dentistry 2003;13:98-105.

Chapter 2
Risk Factors Associated with Dental Erosion

Aim

To summarise the risk factors thought to be associated with dental erosion.

Outcome

After reading this chapter the practitioner should have an understanding of:
- a wide range of intrinsic and extrinsic factors that increase the risk of dental erosion developing
- the different forms of vomiting, and their aetiology, that may produce dental erosion
- the common eating disorders that may result in dental erosion
- the protective role of saliva
- behaviour that increases the risk of dental erosion developing
- the importance of a holistic and individual approach to the management of patients with dental erosion.

The Risk Factors

Exposure of the teeth to acid increases the risk of dental erosion developing. The source of the acid may be either intrinsic (from within the body) or extrinsic (from outwith the body). Extrinsic factors are wide-ranging and include dietary, environmental, medicaments' and lifestyle agents. Figure 2-1 summarises the main risk factors.

The Intrinsic Factors
Any condition or behaviour that results in acid from the gastrointestinal tract coming into contact with the teeth constitutes an intrinsic factor or a breakdown in the protective effects of saliva.

Gastric contents may reach the oral cavity in a variety of ways:
- vomiting – the forceful expulsion of gastric contents through the mouth. The dentist should be aware that where this occurs frequently an organic or psychosomatic disorder may be the cause. These are summarised in Table 2-1.

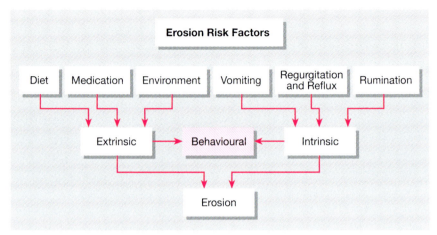

Fig 2-1 The main risk factors for erosion.

- regurgitation and reflux – these differ from vomiting as there is a lack of diaphragmatic muscular contraction, and a relatively small quantity of material is ejected. They are generally associated with increased gastric volume and pressure and could be a sign of an incompetent cardiac sphincter.
- rumination – this may be considered to be a special form of regurgitation. Gastric contents are regurgitated, chewed and reswallowed. This may well be considered a variant of normal behaviour and is probably more common than reported. The social unacceptability of the practice probably inhibits disclosure.

Vomiting and its variants play a significant role in a variety of eating disorders.

Eating disorders
These may be defined as a persistent disturbance of eating behaviour or behaviour intended to control weight that significantly impairs physical health or psychosocial functioning and is not secondary to a general medical condition or another psychiatric disorder. In modern western society it is believed such disorders are on the increase. Four principal types are described currently:
- anorexia nervosa (AN)
- bulimia nervosa (BN)
- eating disorders not otherwise specified (EDNOS)
- binge-eating disorder (BED)

Table 2-1 **Causes of vomiting**

Causes

Disorders of the alimentary tract
- peptic ulcer, chronic gastritis
- disordered gastrointestinal motility (postvagotomy, diabetes, idiopathic gastroparesis)
- intestinal obstruction (e.g. adhesions, malignancy, hernia, volvulus)
- infections of the intestinal tract (gastroenteritis, pancreatitis, hepatitis, cholecystitis, cholangitis)

Central nervous system disorders with increased intracranial pressure
(e.g. encephalitis, neoplasms, hydrocephalus)

Neurological disorders
- migraine headaches
- tabetic crisis
- diabetic or alcoholic polyneuropathia
- disorders of labyrinthine apparatus (e.g. Méniere's disease, benign recurrent vertigo)

Metabolic and endocrine disorders
- uremia
- diabetic ketoacidosis
- hypo-, hyperparathyroidism
- hyperthyroid crisis
- adrenal insufficiency
- pregnancy (hyperemesis gravidarum)

Side-effect of drugs
- central emetic effect (e.g. digitalis, estrogens, chemotherapeutic agents, emetine, histamine, beta blockers, tetracycline, levodopa, opioids)
- gastric irritation with secondary effect of vomiting (e.g. alcohol, salicylates, aminophylline, ipecacuahnha, ferrous sulfate, potassium chloride, diuretics)

Psychosomatic disorders
- stress-induced psychogenic vomiting
- eating disorders (anorexia nervosa, bulimia nervosa)

★ Reproduced from Scheutzel P. Etiology of dental erosion – intrinsic factors. European Journal of Oral Sciences 1995;104:178-190, by kind permission of the Editor, Journal of Oral Sciences.

Anorexia nervosa (AN) – although commonly believed to be a disease of the modern age, was first described independently in literature published during the 1870s by the Englishman Sir William Gull and Frenchman Ernest-Charles Lasegue. The term is derived from the greek orexis, meaning a nervous loss of appetite. It manifests as an aversion to food resulting from a complex interaction between biological, social, individual and family factors, leading to severe weight loss. Its prevalence is of the order of 0.1-1% of young females, with the average age of presentation being 16 years old. Incidence (the number of new cases in the population over one year) is estimated to be seven per 100,000. In general, affected individuals look thin and are more than 15% below ideal body weight. Two subtypes of this condition have been identified: restricting – where weight loss is accomplished primarily by either fasting or excessive exercise, or binge/purge – where loss of weight is achieved with self-induced vomiting or excessive exercise or by the misuse of laxatives, diuretics or enemas. Sufferers display a fear of gaining weight or becoming fat and have disturbed perceptions of their own body shape and size. With an obsession of self-image, there is a relentless pursuit of thinness. This is accompanied by amenorrhea and psychological disturbances.

The duration of the condition is up to six years. Significant mortality (4–20%) is associated with anorexia nervosa, given its medical complications and predisposition to suicide. The level of suicide risk is lower than with bulimia nervosa. Interestingly, a previous history of anorexia nervosa is considered to be a risk factor for the development of bulimia in later life.

Bulimia nervosa (BN) – the term is derived from the Greek bous (head of cattle) and limos (hunger) meaning literally appetite of an ox. It manifests as recurrent episodes of binge eating followed by inappropriate behaviours, such as self-induced vomiting or excessive exercise to avoid weight gain. It is a more common condition than anorexia, with a prevalence of 1-2% for adolescent girls and 0.1% for young men. Its incidence is of the order of eight to 14 cases per 100,000. The average age of presentation is 25 years. Affected individuals are less readily identifiable from their outward appearance, compared to those with anorexia nervosa, being within 10% of their physiological ideal weight. They may even be slightly overweight. Dentists may therefore be the first health professionals to detect this condition by picking up on the early signs of erosive tooth surface loss as they conduct an unconnected dental examination. Two forms of this condition have been described: purging – where body weight is controlled by self- induced vomiting, with a heightened chance of medical complication as a result of disturbances in the bodies electrolytes,

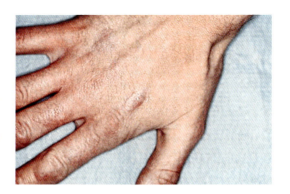

Fig 2-2 Russell's sign – callous formation on the back of the hand used to induce vomiting by a male patient (reproduced by kind permission of the Editor of the British Dental Journal and Dr A Milosevic).

notably reduced sodium (Na) and potassium (K) and increased phosphorus (P) and magnesium (Mg); non-purging – where body weight is controlled by various permutations of excessive exercise and fasting.

Sufferers have a preoccupation with eating and are overly concerned with body weight and shape. Although the associated suicide risk is greater than with anorexia nervosa, a better recovery outcome (up to 80%) is reported. Death is a rare consequence affecting only 0.3% of cases.

An emerging sub-variant is uni/multi-impulsive bulimia where, in addition to the above behaviours, individuals engage in drug abuse, shoplifting and aberrant sexual practices.

Eating disorders not otherwise specified (EDNOS) – the diagnostic criteria for both anorexia nervosa and bulimia are stringent. As a consequence not all patients will meet all the necessary criteria for these conditions although having symptoms severe enough to qualify as suffering from a clinically significant eating disorder. They are therefore given the diagnosis of EDNOS.

Typically the conditions of AN, BN and EDNOS with self-induced vomiting present with dental erosion primarily affecting upper palatal, occlusal and cervical sites. This may also be accompanied by Russell's sign (Fig 2-2) in which there is callus formation on the back of the hand and fingers. This arises from repeatedly putting the hand in the back of the mouth to induce vomiting.

Figure 2-3 summarises the salient features of Anorexia Nervosa and Bulimia Nervosa.

	Anorexia Nervosa	Bulimia Nervosa
Prevalence	0.1 to 1% (♀)	1–2% (♀), 0.1% (♂)
Incidence	7 per 100,000	8–14 per 100,000
Average Age at Presentation (years)	16	25
Duration (years)	6	–
Mortality	4–20%	0.3%
Suicide Risk	lower than BN	greater than AN

Fig 2-3 Comparison of Anorexia and Bulimia Nervosa.

Binge-eating disorder (BED) – a condition that to date is poorly understood. Its prevalence is of the order of 1% affecting males and females equally. Such individuals binge eat to excess but demonstrate no compensatory behaviour to avoid weight gain. They therefore outwardly appear to be overweight or obese. Such individuals by virtue of their size may be considered more prone to acid reflux.

What are the risk factors for anorexia/bulimia?
a) Genetic/family – a family history of either condition increases the likelihood of developing either anorexia nervosa or bulimia. In the case of anorexia the increased risk level is thought to be of the order of seven to 20 times. Research into genetic susceptibility has focused on physiological mechanisms that regulate either food intake (serotonin) or body weight (leptin, melanocortin receptor, oestrogen receptor). Of these the serotonergic pathway is thought to be the most likely. Sufferers of both AN and BN have elevated serotonin metabolites in their cerebrospinal fluid. This is thought by some to correlate directly with the severity of the symptoms. Interestingly, such raised levels of serotonin are also implicated in obsessive-compulsive spectrum disorders that themselves are a risk factor for the development of AN or BN.
b) Temperamental/personality – traits common to AN and BN are increased levels of harm avoidance and perfectionism. Those with AN are said to be persistent, obsessional and conscientious. Anxiety and mood disorders are associated with BN, together with impulsivity and negative emotionality. A contradiction to the above is the high level of self-injurious behaviour exhibited by some with BN. This may manifest as substance abuse, self-mutilation or even suicide. It is not entirely clear if the described behaviours are predisposing factors or consequences of either AN or BN.

c) Developmental – puberty is considered a risk factor in developing AN. It may be that this condition is a psychological reaction to the changing body.

d) Sociocultural – AN is more prevalent in cultures and societies where thinness is considered beautiful and desirable.

The protective role of saliva

Saliva has a major protective role to play against the development of dental erosion. The erosive effects of dietary acids are lessened by this versatile biological fluid. It both washes away and dilutes foods in the mouth, aiding the formation and subsequent removal of the food bolus by swallowing by virtue of its lubricant properties. Its buffers resist changes in pH arising from food intake and help restore the intraoral pH to neutrality. Effects upon tooth substance of such a pH drop are minimised, as saliva is supersaturated with respect to the appatite crystals of the tooth's surface. This impairs the loss of mineral from the tooth surface by the law of mass action. Conversely, when mineral has been lost, saliva aids the remineralisation of tooth substance by precipitating calcium phosphate under favourable pH conditions. It also bathes the tooth surface in fluoride, which itself inhibits a demineralisation. There is considerable individual variation in these functions, which may account for the variations seen in individuals' susceptibility to dental erosion. These have been exploited by a variety of commercially available test kits and are covered further in Chapter 3.

The Extrinsic Factors

The extrinsic factors associated with dental erosion are fourfold:

- dietary
- medication
- environmental
- behavioural.

They may act either singly or in combination.

Dietary factors

Many foods and beverages are acidic. In fact, the acid content is important for both flavour and taste perception. In addition, in convenience products the level of acid is not only controlled by the manufacturer for these reasons but also to assist product stability and shelf life. In addition to carbonated beverages and citric fruit juices a wide variety of other foods and drinks have been associated with the development of dental erosion. These include sports drinks, wines and cider. Healthy lifestyle foods such as certain herbal teas, yoghurts, fruits and berries together with salad dress-

Table 2-2 **The titratable acidity of a number of foods and beverages**

Food/Drink	Titratable acidity
Orange Hooch	23.1 (Range 22.5-23.8)
Apple Hooch	15.4 (Range 15.2-15.7)
Woodpecker Cider	14.54 (0.53)
Raspberry, cranberry and elderflower tea	23.36 (1.89)
Orange juice	21.4 (0.09)
Tea	3.54 (0.46)

⋆ These are the mean volumes, and standard deviation of the observations (except where stated otherwise) of the volume of 0.1 molar sodium hydroxide required to raise the pH of 20ml of the food/drink to neutrality.

ings and vinegar conserves may produce erosion if consumed in excess. It should be stressed that it is not the pH of food or drink that is believed to determine the erosive potential, but the titratable acidity – sometimes also termed neutralisable acidity. It is considered that the higher this quantity is the more potentially erosive a product is. Titratable acidity is the volume of alkali (typically 0.1 molar sodium hydroxide) required to raise the pH of a standardised volume of a beverage (typically 25ml) to pH 7. This is illustrated for a variety of foods and beverages in Table 2-2. Values for a range of carbonated drinks are contained in Table 3-3. Erosive potential may be demonstrated to a patient as both an aid to diagnosis and to reinforce patient education (see Chapter 3 under 'special investigations'). Care must be exercised in extrapolating the results of such a simple laboratory-based test to the clinical situation, however, as it does not reflect the biological compensatory mechanisms of the oral cavity that display considerable variation in effectiveness. The quantity, duration and frequency of intake of acidic foods and drinks are important factors to consider in assessing the likelihood of a food or beverage being responsible for the dental erosion observed in a patient. Excessive and frequent

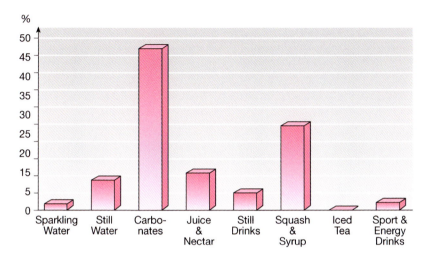

Fig 2-4 Percentage UK Soft Drink Market Share according to Drink Type for 2003 (Data Source: Canadean & Canmakers Report, 2004).

consumption are most likely to produce erosion in a susceptible individual. Those who sip a carbonated beverage over a long period of time increase the length of time the salivary pH is below the critical pH, compared to those who consume it relatively quickly. It should also be borne in mind that the excessive consumption of such drinks to quench thirst, in an apparently well individual, may be a sign of undiagnosed diabetes. In recent years there has been a very large increase in the sales of such drinks. This has been attributed to the increased availability and affordable price of a greatly expanded range of heavily marketed drinks. Although the annual consumption of soft drinks in the UK is 235 litres per person, carbonates account for only 47% of this (Fig 2-4). The UK annual consumption of carbonated drinks, per head of population, is around 99 litres which is approximately half that in the USA, but greater than in other European countries (Fig 2-5).

Medication
Any medicament that has both a low pH and high titratable acidity that comes into contact with the teeth has the potential to produce dental erosion. The frequency and duration of consumption should be considered together with the form in which the medicament comes. Frequent intakes over a lengthy course of medication are most likely to produce erosion. Those who take

13

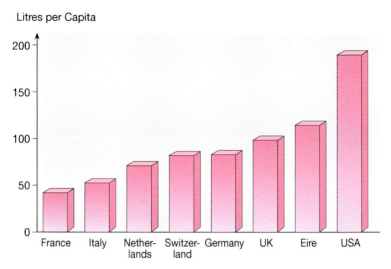

Fig 2-5 Consumption of carbonated soft drinks in 2003 according to country (Data Source: Can Makers Report 2004).

chewable aspirin tablets have a greater likelihood of dental erosion than those who swallow such tablets directly. Individuals with alchorhydria, receiving liquid hydrochloric acid orally in their treatment, are at greater risk of erosion than those who take it in capsulated form. Other medicaments reported to be associated with erosion include both iron tonics and vitamin C tablets. It should also be borne in mind that acidic salivary flow stimulants and salivary substitutes containing citric or malic acid have been linked to erosion. These products are generally taken by individuals whose own protective mechanism against erosion is compromised given a lack of saliva. It has also been suggested that reduced salivary flow in those using inhalers to control asthma may account for the reported higher incidence of dental erosion in such individuals. This has not been substantiated.

Environmental
With today's more stringent Health and Safety legislation compared to previous years it is less likely that workers will be exposed to an acidic working environment than was formally the case. Many industrial processes produce or use nitric, sulphuric or hydrochloric acids. Traditionally, those working with dynamite and munitions, in battery manufacture, printing, galvanising plants and fertiliser manufacturer were said to be more prone to develop den-

tal erosion. Professional wine tasters are also at risk given the repeated contact of acidic wine with the teeth as they perform their work.

Those who regularly swim in chlorinated swimming pools may be at greater risk of developing erosion in particular if the pool pH is not monitored and carefully maintained. The gas chlorination of swimming pools produces hydrochloric acid that must be neutralised and buffered to maintain a safe pool pH. This requires regular monitoring by the pool attendant.

Behavioural
Any behaviour that involves the excessive consumption of acidic foods and drinks may lead to the development of dental erosion. It is accepted that a healthier lifestyle involves both regular exercise and the consumption of plenty fruits and vegetables. This is sound advice but should not be taken to extremes.

Strenuous sporting activities reduce the level of saliva flow, increase the loss of body fluids and consume energy. Subsequently there is the need to both quench the thirst and satisfy hunger. Often individuals following exercise consume low pH sugar containing carbonated drinks which, combined with the reduced salivary flow, risk eroding the dentition. A further acidic challenge to the teeth arises from the increased potential for acid reflux during and following exercise.

Diets in which the level of intake of acidic 'healthier foods' is taken to extremes may bring about dental erosion. In this regard the consumption of large quantities of citric fruits, yoghurts, acidic fruit and herbal teas may be damaging to the teeth. An excessive consumption of citric fruit may form part of a weight reduction plan, indicating perhaps a degree of dissatisfaction with the present lifestyle. It is generally believed that a vegetarian diet may increase the chances of developing erosion. Vegetables contain many acids which may be damaging if consumed in excess.

By definition dental erosion occurs in the absence of plaque. Indeed, the presence of plaque in the form of pellicle may be protective against the development of dental erosion. Some would argue that the modern day obsession of cleanliness, manifesting in the vigorous use of dentifrices and mouth rinses, removes the protective pellicle and increases susceptibility to erosion. Another factor to consider is the repeated use of home bleaching kits by the patient in the quest for 'perfect' white teeth. This can be damaging to the enamel over a prolonged period of use, in particular, when combined with over zealous brushing.

In specific relation to 'youth culture' it is not uncommon, within, for example, a student population, to observe dental erosion associated with the consumption of acidic high-caffeine energy drinks commonly mixed with vodka. The typical pattern of activity may be to study during the early part of the evening, whilst perhaps sharing a bottle of wine, and then go out to socialise until late sustained by a number of cans of such a drink with or without alcohol.

Those who frequently attend raves and take the designer drug ecstasy (3, 4 methaylene dioxy-methamphetamine) may exhibit dental erosion as a consequence of their excessive consumption of acidic drinks. Such thirst results from a combination of the dry mouth effect of the drug and the physical activity of the rave. In this instance damage to the teeth is most often the combined effects of both erosion and attrition.

Young adults who indulge in frequent alcoholic binges may exhibit erosion. Such binges are often followed by episodes of vomiting. In general 'booze bingers' are open about such activities. Of greater concern however, are those who may have developed chronic alcoholism that have not yet recognised, let alone accepted, they have a problem. Alcoholics tend to be secretive about their habit and confirmation is difficult. The application of the CAGE questionnaire may be helpful in eliciting such information (see Chapter 3 – under Special Investigations) and the dentist should seek to arrange professional help where consent is given.

Further Reading

Chadwick R G, Mitchell H L, Manton S L, Ward S, Ogston S and Brown R Maxillary incisor palatal erosion: no correlation with dietary variables? J Clin Pediatr Dent 2005;29:157-164.

Klein D. A. and Walsh T. B. Eating disorders: clinical features and pathophysiology. Physiology and Behaviour 2004;81:359-374.

Scheutzel P. Etiology of dental erosion – intrinsic factors. European Journal of Oral Sciences 1996;104:178-190.

Zero D.T Etiology of dental erosion – extrinsic factors. European Journal of Oral Sciences 1996;104:241-244.

Chapter 3
Formulating a Management Strategy

Aim

To outline a systematic approach to history taking, examining, investigating, assimilating and arriving at a diagnosis so that a management strategy, tailored to the individual patient, may be formulated.

Outcome

After reading this chapter the practitioner should have an understanding of:
- what to look out for in both a patient's history and medical history
- what to look out for when conducting both an intraoral and extraoral examination
- the importance of the patients' expectations
- the application of some useful special investigations (Dietary survey tools, Radiographic examination, Study models and intraoral radiographs, salivary tests)
- behaviour that increases the risk of dental erosion developing
- the importance of a holistic and individual approach to the management of patients with dental erosion

Making the Diagnosis

The development of dental erosion is insidious. Often it is a member of the dental team who will be the first to discover that the patient has this condition. It is generally not until the integrity of the enamel is breached that a patient will report any symptoms, such as sensitivity of the affected teeth to hot or cold. It is therefore important that the early signs are recognised and acted upon, in consultation with the patient, if the condition is to be prevented from progressing further.

Making a definitive diagnosis to develop a management strategy, tailored to the individual patients needs, involves four principal components:
- History taking
- Acquisition of the medical history
- An extra- and intraoral examination
- Determining the patients' expectations.

Each may act as a trigger for a special investigation to acquire further information to assist in the development of the management strategy.

History Taking

It is important to elicite from the patient when and for how long they have been aware of the problem. Typically, the patient will report chipping of the incisal edges, fracture of teeth and alterations in the appearance of anterior teeth, such as greying of the incisal edge following an alteration in translucency as a result of loss of palatal tooth substance. Where dentine has become exposed, pain or sensitivity of the teeth may be reported. This could be upon exposure to hot and cold drinks or even on toothbrushing following the intake of an acidic food.

Acquisition of the Medical History

A comprehensive medical history should always be obtained and recorded. With specific reference to dental erosion, it is important to establish any potential source of intrinsic acid. This could be as a result of an undiagnosed level of gastro-oesophageal reflux, reported by the patient as heartburn or indigestion, arising from either an underlying medical condition (Table 3-1) or as a side-effect of medication (Table 3-2).

Extraoral and Intraoral Examination

Extraoral – the outward appearance of the patient as they enter the surgery can tell much information - for example, does the patient look under- or overweight? It is also useful to look at the hands to see if a callous on the back of the hand and fingers is present. This is known as Russell's Sign (see Fig 2-2) and may indicate the use of fingers to induce vomiting in a patient with an eating disorder.

Intraorally – the early signs of erosion include the loss of tooth surface characteristics generally from plaque-free sites. Any tooth morphological sharp angles appear rounded and the enamel surface may appear smooth and polished. This may be accompanied by an alteration in the optical properties of the affected surface. As the condition progresses the enamel becomes thinner ultimately resulting in exposure of areas of the underlying dentine. Once exposed, the dentine surface becomes grooved or may even display cupping such as seen on the cusp tips of the affected molars (Fig 3-1). The patient may then experience sensitivity upon exposure to hot and cold. As the enamel progressively thins, it displays increased translucency and may ultimately fracture. Such alterations in the appearance of the anterior teeth do not go unnoticed by the patient.

Table 3-1 **Causes of gastroesophageal reflux and regurgitation**

Causes

Incompetence of the gastroesophageal sphincter

Primary
• idiopathic with or without hiatus hernia secondary

Secondary
• impairment of the gastroesophageal sphincter by progressive systemic sclerosis, mixed connective tissue disease, and neurogenic disorders (e.g. diabetic and alcoholic polyneuropathia)
• destruction of the sphincter by surgical resection, myotomie, ballon dilatation or esophagitis
• neurohormonal induced decrease of gastroesophageal sphincter pressure by drugs (e.g. beta-adrenergics, serotonin, cholecystokinin, diazepam, glukagon), increased estrogen and progesterone (luteal phase of menstrual cycle, pregnancy, intake of oral contraceptives), diet (fatty meals, peppermint, chocolate, coffee, alcohol) or smoking

Increased intraabdominal pressure
• obesity
• pregnancy
• ascites

Increased intragastric volume
• after meals
• pyloric spasm
• obstruction due to peptic ulcer, gastroparesis
• gastric stasis syndrome

★ Reproduced from Scheutzel P. Etiology of dental erosion – intrinsic factors. European Journal of Oral Sciences 1995;104:178-190, by kind permission of the Editor, Journal of Oral Sciences.

Any restorations of either amalgam or resin composite – materials that are inert to the erosive process, appear to sit proud relative to the surrounding tooth structure as this erodes away. This is termed submargination (Fig 3-

Table 3–2 **List of drugs that may cause vomiting as a side-effect**

List of drugs

Anorectics
Fenfluramine
Amfepramone
Piracetam
Phendimetrazine
Mazindol

Antiallergic drugs and antitussives
Clofedanol
Cranoglycate disodium
Letosteine

Antibiotics
Tetracyclines

Anticonvulsants
Progabide
γ-vinyl-GABA
Buprenorphine

Antifungal drugs
Nystatin

Drugs acting on the peripheral circulation
Buphenine
Co-dergocrine
Isoxsuprine

Drugs affecting autonomic function or the extrapyramidal system
Amantadine
Carbidopa
Dopamine
Ergometrine
Ergotamine
Mesulergine
Piribedil
Serotonin
Tyrosine

Drugs increasing dopamine activity
Amantadine

Drugs of abuse
Cannabis nutmeg

Opioid analgesics
Alfentanil
Buprenorphine
Buturphanol
Ciramadol
Conorfone
Cyclazocine
Dezocine
Nalbuphine
Naloxone
Naltrexone
Pentazocine
Sufentanil
Tramadol

Opioid agonists
Alfentamil
Amantadine
Butorphanol
Ciramadol

Antihypertensive drugs
Nitroprusside
Clonidine

Anti-inflammatory analgesics and drugs used in gout
Ibuprofen
Indometacin
Phenylbutazone
Piroxicam

Antiprotozoal drugs
Iodoquinol
Emetine

Antipyretic analgesics
Acetylsalicylic acid and related compounds

Central nervous system stimulants
Caffeine
Theophylline and related substances
Doxapram
Euprofylline
Lobeline

Lysergide tetrahydrocannabiol

Gastrointestinal drugs
Salazosulfapyridine
Mercaptamine
Fentagastrin
Loperamide

General anesthetics
Cyclopropane
Isoflurane

Hypnotics and sedatives
Benzodiazepines
Chloralhydrate
Ethylchlorrynol
Methaqualone

Immunomodulating agents
Preabanil
Lithium

Metals
Gallium nitrate
Gold salts
Iron salts

Positive inotropic drugs and drugs used in dysarrhythmias
Aprindine
Bretylium
Digitalis glycosides
Flecainide
Lorcainide
Tocainide

Prostaglandins
Sex hormones
Estrogens
Tamoxifen

Stimulant and anorectic agents
Cocaine
Methylphenidate

Tricyclic antidepressants
Fluoxetine
Fluvoxamine
Tryptophan
Viloxazine

Nikethamide
Proproxyphylline

Cytostatic and immunosuppressive drugs
Diuretics
Spironolactone
Thiazide diuretics
triamterene

Selenium
Zinc

Metal antagonists
Dimercaprol

★ Reproduced from Scheutzel P. Etiology of dental erosion – intrinsic factors. European Journal of Oral Sciences 1995;104:178-190, by kind permission of the Editor, Journal of Oral Sciences.

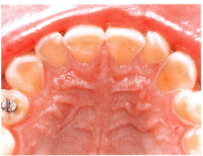

Fig 3-1 Cupping of the cusp tips of molars as a result of erosion.

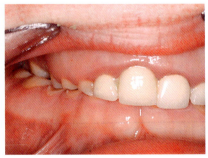

Fig 3-2 Submargination of an amalgam restoration in the upper right first premolar.

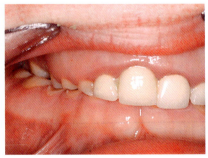

Fig 3-3 Alveolar overgrowth in a patient with severe tooth surface loss attributed to a combination of erosion and bruxism.

2). If no other mechanism of tooth surface loss is involved (such as abrasion or attrition) there is a lack of faceting.

Young adults affected by erosion are generally both concerned about the appearance of their anterior teeth and distressed about the sensitivity. In addition, they are worried about the longevity of their dentition. As the loss of tooth substance continues loss of vitality and apical pathology may result.

As tooth tissue is lost there may be either compensatory tooth movement or alveolar growth (Fig 3-3) to maintain the occlusal vertical dimension (OVD). On the other hand, if the rate of loss exceeds these compensatory mechanisms then OVD may be reduced. This has important consequences if restoration is to be undertaken.

Determining the Patient's Expectations

As dental erosion tends to affect young adults, many of who are concerned about self image, it is important to determine what they wish for any dental intervention. Do they simply want to prevent further tooth surface loss, or wish to regain the tissue that has been lost in the process, or even improve upon their past dental appearance? This information is essential to determine before embarking upon any management strategy to ensure that what is to be achieved coincides with the patients expectations. This of course may not be possible, and the patient should be informed of this from the outset.

In working through these four stages a variety of investigations may be of assistance. These include:

- dietary survey supported by laboratory analysis
- radiographic examination
- study models and intra oral photographs
- salivary tests

Special Investigations

Dietary survey – many approaches to the dietary survey are available, ranging from structured forms to a blank sheet of paper. Many prefer the latter due to its simplicity. It is important to stress to the patient that they should be honest in writing down their dietary intake, as you wish to help them. False entries invalidate the process and render it a futile exercise. When asking patients to record for one week when and what they eat and drink, avoid the temptation of telling them what you are looking for. At the next visit

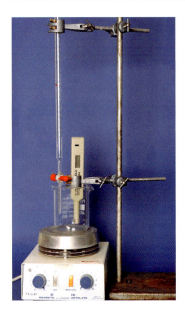

Fig 3-4 Apparatus required to determine the titratable acidity.

highlight the acid foods and drinks with a highlighter pen and, if found to be consumed frequently, offer appropriate advice. Sometimes a drink may be encountered about which the erosive potential is unknown. For those minded to assist their patients in understanding the cause of their erosion it is comparatively simple to determine the erosive potential of a sample by determining its titratable acidity.

Determination of titratable acidity - Relatively inexpensive items of equipment are required – retort stand, burette, reagent beakers, pH meter and a supply of a solution of 0.1 M sodium hydroxide (Fig 3-4). The sodium hydroxide could be made up either by a chemist or by the dentist. A total of 25ml of the drink should be placed in the beaker and its pH recorded. By making small additions of 0.1 M sodium hydroxide from burette into the drink, whilst agitating the beaker to aid mixing, determine the required volume of sodium hydroxide to raise the pH to 7. This is the titratable acidity. Typical values of this are contained in Table 3-3 for a wide variety of carbonated drinks. It is not an exact science. The value will depend upon how rapidly the titration is carried out from opening the bottle/can. This is because the carbon dioxide in the opened drink is gradually lost to the atmosphere.

Table 3-3 **The titratable acidity of a wide variety of carbonated drinks**

Product	Mean titratable acidity	S.D.
Ribena Toothkind – Tropical Orange	6.48	0.40
Dr Pepper	7.60	0.87
Pepsi – Diet	7.66	0.98
Coke – Diet	7.76	0.52
Coke – Cherry	7.96	0.92
Coke – Diet Caffeine Free	8.02	0.85
Pepsi Max	9.34	0.47
Dr Pepper – Diet	9.42	0.81
Coca-Cola	9.52	0.81
Pepsi	9.68	0.93
Ribena Blackcurrant Juice Drink	12.26	1.03
Tizer	12.26	1.55
Vimto – Light	13.36	1.15
Barr Lemonade	13.98	1.67
Barr Diet IRN-Bru	13.98	1.30
Panda Pops – Lemonade	14.58	1.32
Sprite – Light	17.30	1.62
Sprite	17.58	1.58

7-Up	17.86	1.64
Panda Pops – Strawberry Jelly & Ice Cream	18.04	1.72
Schweppes Lemonade – Diet	18.56	2.06
Lucozade Sport	19.14	1.70
Tango Apple – Diet	19.48	2.19
Schweppes Lemonade	19.62	2.03
Tango Cherry – Diet	19.88	1.63
Tango Apple	20.53	2.04
Rio – Florida	21.80	2.30
Lipovitan B3	22.22	2.11
Fanta Orange – Diet	22.60	1.71
Fanta Orange	22.64	1.76
Tango – New Diet Tropical	22.98	2.15
Lilt – Diet Totally Tropical	23.22	1.98
7-Up Light	23.64	0.38
Solstis – Lucozade Fast Stimulation for Body & Mind	23.86	2.49
Red Devil Energy Drink	24.62	1.78
Tango – Diet Orange	25.22	2.05
Red Bull	33.2	3.08

★ Mean titratable acidity is the mean volume of 0.1 molar sodium hydroxide, for five 25 ml samples of each drink, required to raise the pH to 7.0.

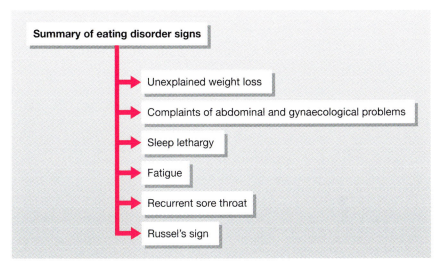

Fig 3-5 Eating disorder signs.

In recording the patients history or whilst analysing the dietary survey, suspicion may be raised as to whether a patient has an eating disorder or an alcohol problem. In such circumstances the application of a screening questionnaire may be helpful.

Screening for eating disorders – Denial and shame are strongly associated with these disorders. As a result, many sufferers attempt to conceal such conditions or present with other symptoms. The dentist should be aware that unexplained weight loss, complaints of abdominal and gynaecological problems or sleep lethargy and fatigue may be signs of an eating disorder (Fig 3-5). In addition, sufferers may have a sore throat from recurrent vomiting, together with Russell's sign (see Fig 2-2). The presence of dental erosion primarily affecting palatal, occlusal and cervical sites may be the first outward sign that an individual has an eating disorder. The dentist may thus be the first healthcare professional to become aware of the condition and should liaise with the medical practitioner, with the consent of the patient. Helpful tools in making an early diagnosis include a dietary history, knowledge of ideal height and weight charts (see Figs 3-6 and 3-7) together with the application of the SCOFF questionnaire (Table 3-4). This consists of a serious of five questions that address the core features of AN and BN. One point is awarded for every yes; a score of > 2 indicates a likely case of AN or BN.

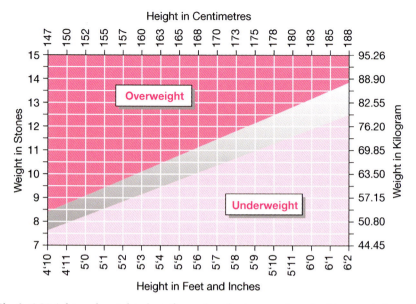

Fig 3-6 Height and weight chart for male – basis reproduced with permission of www.weightlossresources.co.uk

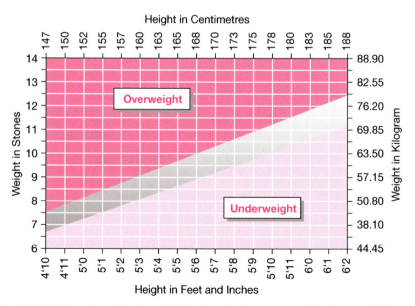

Fig 3-7 Height and weight chart for female – basis reproduced with permission of www.weightlossresources.co.uk

28

Table 3-4 **The SCOFF questionnaire**

SCOFF questionnaire
1. Do you make yourself Sick because you feel uncomfortably full? 2. Do you worry you have lost Control over how much you eat? 3. Have you recently lost more than One stone in a three-month period? 4. Do you believe yourself to be Fat when others say you are too thin? 5. Would you say Food dominates your life?

★ One point for every 'YES' score; a score of > 2 indicates a likely case of AN or Bulimia.

It should be emphasised that it is designed to raise suspicion of a likely case, rather than to diagnose.

Screening for alcoholism – In general young adults who engage in binge drinking are open about their activities. There are also those who may have developed chronic alcoholism, but have not recognised that they have a problem. These individuals tend to be more secretive about their activities. In such circumstances the application of the CAGE questionnaire may be of help. This consists of a series of four questions (Table 3-5) that are asked verbally. A positive response is not diagnostic of alcoholism, but it is generally considered that two such responses should alert the interviewer to the likelihood of the patient suffering from alcoholism.

Radiographic examination – periapical films are helpful to establish the apical status of teeth that have been eroded and for determining the level of bone support (Fig 3-8). Bitewing films will assist in the diagnosis of approximal caries. This is of particular importance for those whose erosion is linked to an eating disorder such as BN (Fig 3-9). A panoramic image/view (Fig 3-10) is also of assistance where extensive tooth destruction has occurred as a result of both caries and erosion. Sometimes, due to self shame concerning their dental appearance, some individuals do not seek dental care until they are in pain.

Study models and intraoral photographs – these are of particular help to assess the impact of preventive advice upon the erosive process. Comparison of

Table 3-5 **The CAGE questionnaire**

CAGE questionnaire

1. Have you ever felt you ought to Cut down on your drinking?
2. Have people Annoyed you by criticising your drinking?
3. Have you ever felt bad or Guilty about your drinking?
4. Have you ever had a drink first thing in the morning to steady your nerves or get rid of a hangover (Eye-opener)?

★ Reproduced from Ewing JA. Detecting alcoholism – the CAGE questionnaire. Journal of the American Association 1984;252:1905-1907). By kind permission from the Editor of the Journal of The American Medical Association. Copyright © 1984, American Medical Association. All rights reserved.

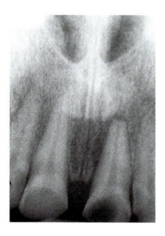

Fig 3-8 Periapical radiograph of UR1 UL1 – Both teeth demonstrate severe palatal loss of tooth substance. That on UL1 has resulted in pulpal exposure and periapical pathology.

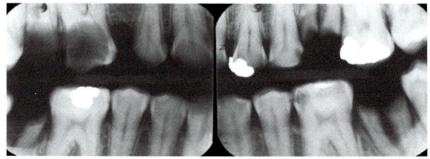

Fig 3-9 Bitewing radiographs of a bulimic patient.

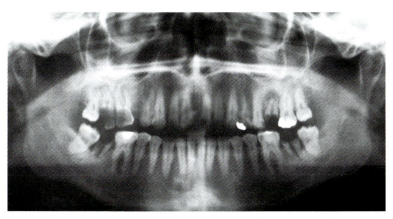

Fig 3-10 DPT of patient who in the past secretly suffered from bulimia and only now has summoned up courage to seek dental help.

baseline models and photographs with a patient directly or a more recent set of study models, at some stage in the future can establish if the condition has progressed. In general, sequential casts allow a much clearer assessment of the extent of wear. They also serve as a valuable patient motivational and educational aid. They can also form the basis of a diagnostic wax up to discuss possible treatment options (Fig 3-11). When recording these in alginate the detail of occlusal surface capture may be optimised by rubbing unset alginate onto these surfaces prior to seating the loaded impression tray.

Salivary tests – undoubtedly, individual susceptibility to the erosive process is of importance in determining its onset and progression. Saliva is a major protective factor against the erosive process. A variety of commercial testing

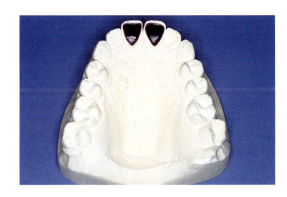

Fig 3-11 Diagnostic wax up of palatal veneers on UR1 and UL1 to facilitate patient discussion.

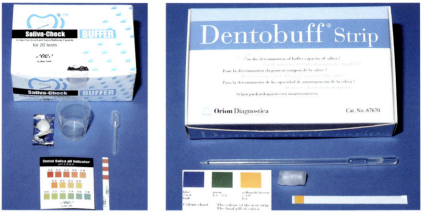

Fig 3-12 Examples of commercially available testing kits to assay the characteristics of a patient's saliva, including buffering power.

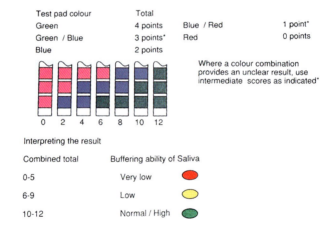

Fig 3-13 Standard chart for buffering power as included in the GC Saliva-Check testing kit.

kits are available to determine the salivary flow rates and buffering capacities of whole mouth saliva in both the resting and stimulated states (Fig 3-12). Flow rate is determined by the collection of saliva in a measuring cup over a defined time period. Buffering capacity is assessed by applying a small quantity of a collected saliva to a chemical testing strip. The colour change following application to the strip relative to a standard chart, indicates the buffering power (Fig 3-13). Stimulated saliva flow is elicited by the patient chewing upon the supplied block of paraffin wax for a defined period of time while expectorating the accumulated fluid into a measuring cup. Normal salivary flow rates are 0.3ml/min when resting and 1.75ml/min in the stimulated state. Low buffering capacity and flow rate indicate a greater erosion risk and advice should be given to the patient to minimise this. This should include following acidic intake with a glass of water to aid clearance and finishing each meal with a neutral salivary stimulant, such as cheese, to promote salivary flow.

Further Reading

Ewing JA. Detecting alcoholism – The CAGE questionnaire. Journal of the American Medical Association 1984;252:1905-1907.

Morgan JF, Reid F, Lacy JH. The SCOFF questionnaire: assessment of a new screening tool for eating disorders. British Medical Journal 1999;319:1467-1468.

Chapter 4
Preventive Measures

Aim

To appreciate that dental erosion may be prevented from occurring or progressing further and, as a result, does not always require restorative operative intervention.

Outcome

After reading this chapter the practitioner should have an understanding of:
- a range of preventive advice to counter the development/progression of dental erosion
- the level of the public's knowledge and understanding concerning dental erosion
- the importance of the early recognition of dental erosion from both a dental and holistic health care perspective
- the implications of different forms of restorative treatment for dental erosion and the need to keep avenues open for future treatment needs
- how to create space for dental restorations
- the importance of long term follow-up.

Prevention and Treatment

The management of dental erosion in the young adult presents a number of dilemmas to the dentist. The institution of preventive measures has to be weighed against the risk of further loss of tooth substance, complicating or precluding restoration. Any operative intervention needs to be carefully considered for it will have to survive many years. Future options for treatment should be kept as open as possible. Any treatment carried out needs to be recoverable when it fails. Furthermore, the potential for meeting the patients' often high aesthetic expectations needs to be carefully explored (Fig 4-1). Such decisions are further complicated by the inevitable changes that may occur in both the habits and psychological status of the patient as they progress through adulthood.

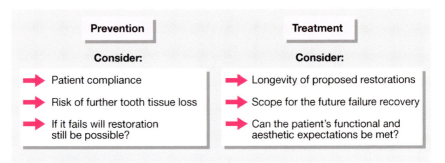

Fig 4-1 Prevention versus treatment.

Prevention

The corner stones of this are:
- education
- early recognition
- risk assessment
- control of further tooth surface loss.

Education

It is essential to actively engage the patient in this process. The success of preventive measures depends greatly upon the active participation of the individual. An early measure of the level of cooperation of the patient is the completion of a dietary diary. Any acidic foods and drinks identified in this by the dental team can serve as a valuable means of initiating a discussion with the patient on the causes and prevention of erosion. This personalises the information given to the patient and promotes a two-way dialogue than the more abstract but true message that acid foods and beverages promote dental erosion. Having caught the imagination of the patient in this way, the opportunity to impart further information should not be lost. This should include advice, where appropriate, to reduce the frequency of acidic intake and to follow such intakes with a rinse of water to aid clearance. Some would also advocate the stimulation of salivary flow following exposure to acid by either chewing sugar-free gum or consuming a neutral food such as cheese. Potential for such action to bring about the remineralisaton of the softened tooth substance should be stressed. It should also be indicated that regular tooth brushing with a fluoride toothpaste both promotes remineralisation and renders the enamel less susceptible to acid attack. Brushing should, however, be delayed until approximately one hour after dietary intake. This is because brushing softened tooth substance

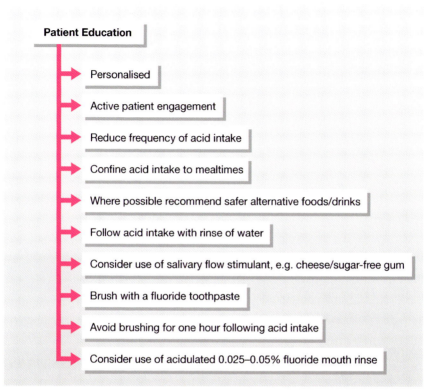

Patient Education

- Personalised
- Active patient engagement
- Reduce frequency of acid intake
- Confine acid intake to mealtimes
- Where possible recommend safer alternative foods/drinks
- Follow acid intake with rinse of water
- Consider use of salivary flow stimulant, e.g. cheese/sugar-free gum
- Brush with a fluoride toothpaste
- Avoid brushing for one hour following acid intake
- Consider use of acidulated 0.025–0.05% fluoride mouth rinse

Fig 4-2 Patient education.

may accelerate the erosive process by simply removing mineralised tissue by the mechanical action of the brushing process. Use of a 0.025 - 0.05% non-acidulated fluoride mouth rinse may also be helpful. These points are summarised in Fig 4-2.

Wherever possible, acid intake should be confined to meal times, and 'safer' alternatives should be indicated to gradually wean a patient of a preferred, but damaging, food or drink. Knowledge of the titratable acidity of various products (see Tables 2-2 and 3-3) or even its determination in the surgery by the dentist (see under Chapter 3 – Special Investigations) in the patients' presence can be helpful in the educative process. Of course, the ideal would be for all patients to discontinue acidic intake, but this is not always considered realistic.

Recent research on public knowledge of erosion indicates confusion. This spans both those who attend a dentist regularly and those who do not. Although being aware of the term dental erosion, those surveyed tend to be under the impression that such damage is due to sugar consumption and not related to acid. A considerable number, however, implicate the consumption of fizzy drinks in the aetiology of erosion. Faced with such confusion, the educative phase of the consultation is of great importance to maximise the chances of success of any preventive measures.

Early recognition
To minimise the impact of the erosive process upon the dentition, members of the dental team should be vigilant to the signs and symptoms of erosion. These are covered in the section on diagnosis. Any early sign should trigger investigation, with both appropriate advice to the patient and the institution of preventive measures.

Risk assessment
The development of dental erosion is more likely when an individual:
- has good oral hygiene – the thinner pellicle confers less protection to the tooth surface upon exposure to acid
- consumes excessive quantities of acidic beverages
- has an eating disorder that results in vomiting
- has a medical disorder that is associated either with gastric reflux or vomiting
- displayed dental erosion as a child.

It is also important to realise that erosion may also be a manifestation of the combined effects of acid intake, softening of the mineralised tooth tissue, compounded further by parafunctional activity such as nocturnal bruxism. This rapidly removes tooth substance, as a result of both mechanical and chemical actions.

Control of further tooth substance loss
This may be achieved by a variety of means either singularly or in combination.
- Dietary modification
- Behaviour modification
- Dental intervention
- Medical intervention.

It is essential that the impact upon the loss of tooth substance of these regimes is monitored. At present only sequential study models have found widespread acceptance for this purpose.

Dietary modification – involves the identification of acidic foods and beverages that are consumed by the patient, followed by their elimination or substitution with 'safer' alternatives in the diet.

Behaviour modification – the patient should be advised to minimise the frequency of intake of acidic foods and preferably confine these to meal times. Acidic intake should be followed by rinsing with water to aid clearance and chewing sugar-free gum to both promote salivary flow and facilitate remineralisation. Brushing should be delayed for approximately one hour after acidic intake so that the mechanical action does not remove softened tooth substance. The use of a fluoridated toothpaste and rinses with a 0.025-0.05% non-acidulated fluoride mouth rinse should also be encouraged to aid remineralisation and render the enamel less acceptable to acid attack.

For those patients whose erosion is as a consequence of vomiting, it is important that the oral pH is raised to avoid further tooth tissue loss. Chewing sugar-free gum and rinsing the mouth with water or milk as soon as possible thereafter is helpful.

Although recently a commercial product (GC-tooth mousse) (Fig 4-3) based upon the milk protein CPP-ACP (casein phosphopeptide-amorphous calcium phosphate) has become available that both creates a so-called protective

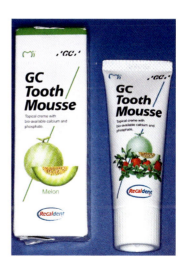

Fig 4-3 GC-tooth mousse – product based upon the milk protein CPP-ACP that is said to both create a protective and 'super' pellicle upon tooth substance.

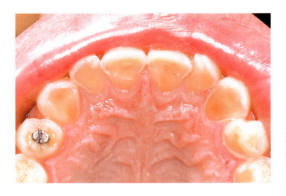

Fig 4-4 Submargination of occlusal amalgam restoration in the UR4 in a patient with palatal tooth surface loss.

and 'super' pellicle upon tooth substance and increases the availability of calcium and phosphate for remineralisation (for both professional and instructed patient application), its efficacy in preventing erosion is as yet unclear.

Dental intervention – as well as the professional application of both fluoride and CPP-ACP (see under behaviour modification) the dentist may also consider replacing failed occlusal restorations and carrying out stain removal from the teeth. Failed occlusal restorations should be replaced so as to preserve the original OVD. Staining should be removed professionally in order to limit the potential for further tooth tissue loss by vigorous and injudicious patient tooth cleaning regimes.

Submargination of dental restorations is commonly seen in cases of dental erosion (Fig 4-4). The restorative material is relatively inert to acid attack and unlike the tooth does not undergo a change in morphology. As a result such restorations appear high relative to the affected tooth substance. Although it is tempting to replace the restoration upon failure to conform with the surrounding eroded tooth structure, this should be resisted. Loss of the occlusal height of the restoration will both disrupt the occlusion, by subsequent tooth migration, and over the course of repeated restoration placement and replacement potentially lead to a reduction in the occlusal vertical dimension of the patient, thereby complicating future restorative work. All such restorations should, when failed, be replaced to the original (high) occlusal height. In this regard the use of adhesively bonded onlay restorations will both maintain the occlusal vertical dimension and protect/cover up the eroded occlusal tooth substance.

Sometimes patients present with tooth surface loss arising from their attempts to improve upon the appearance of the teeth. This may be as a result of excessive use of whitening kits or because more aggressive means of tooth cleansing, such as cotton buds with lemon juice or brillo pads, have been employed. Where possible, professional stain removal can prevent further uncontrolled tooth surface loss occurring by discouraging inappropriate methods of cleaning.

Medical intervention – when any medication a patient may be receiving is thought to induce vomiting, this should be investigated and the patient referred for a possible change in medication. Those medications whose side-effects include vomiting are listed in Table 3-2. It may also be helpful to refer a patient to a physician so that suspected gastric oesophageal reflux may be investigated and treated if found to be appropriate (see Chapter 5, Section 2).

Treatment
The decision to treat can be a difficult one to take and should be taken only after a period of monitoring. Some would argue that unless the erosive process has ceased, definitive restorations should not be provided. Further tooth substance loss will occur around restorations unless the aetiological factors are controlled. Whereas the logic of such a viewpoint is understandable, it does risk further valuable tooth tissue loss that may limit any future potential for restoration. Clearly a balance has to be struck between such viewpoints. In general, therefore, it would be appropriate to treat where (Fig 4-5):

- Any known aetiological risk factors have been minimised by dietary and behavioural modifications and/or medical treatment
- There are symptoms such as dentine hypersensitivity

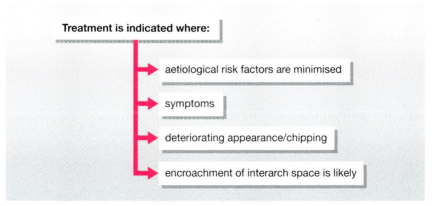

Fig 4-5 Indications for treatment

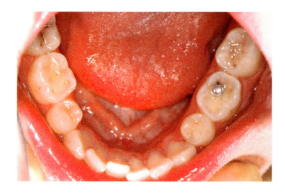

Fig 4-6 Localised occlusal pit on the mesiolingual cusp of the LR6 that was acutely sensitive to acidic foods.

- Due to a loss of tooth substance there is a deterioration in appearance and/or a likelihood of chipping of the tooth
- The tooth tissue loss will lead to an encroachment of space, due to the maintenance of functional contacts by compensatory tooth movement, compromising the future provision of an aesthetic or functional restoration.

Given the inevitable need to replace any restoration in the lifetime of the individual, it is prudent to utilise treatments that involve the minimal sacrifice of tooth structure. This keeps open future more aggressive forms of treatment, such as conventional crownwork, for later in the patients' lifetime. Available treatments include:

- Desensitisation of sensitive exposed dentine
- Control of exacerbating occlusal factors by stabilisation splints
- Adhesive replacement of tooth substance by
  - Occlusal infills or onlays
  - Palatal veneers and labial veneers (singly or in combination)
  - Dentine-bonded crowns.

It is helpful to discuss any such restorative treatment with the patient before proceeding with the aid of both diagnostic wax ups and photographs. This is particularly so given the high aesthetic expectations of many of the affected individuals.

- Desensitisation of sensitive exposed dentine – this is of great value where there is a limited amount of exposed dentine. For example, in either a localised occlusal pit or on proximal surfaces which, although not deep or extensive enough to warrant restoration, is associated with acute dentine hypersensitivity upon exposure to hot, cold or acidic foods (Fig 4-

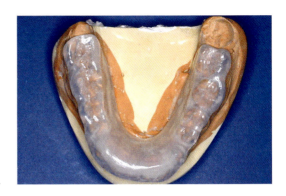

Fig 4-7 A stabilisation splint.

6). Until relatively recently, the only treatments available were the application of fluoride gels and the use of desensitising toothpastes. Neither of these achieve predictable results in either the short or long term. The application, however, of modern dentine-bonding agents to such affected sites offers a predictable and instant treatment. Although this treatment does not generally warrant the application of local anaesthesia, it may be necessary to administer in the more severe circumstances. On applying such agents, great care must be exercised to limit the overspill of the dentine-bonding agent to the gingivae. Many of the available products contain hydroxy ethyl methacrylate (HEMA), which is a very powerful contact allergen. It also penetrates the operating gloves of the dental team. It is therefore good practice to remove the gloves and wash the hands as soon as possible after use if HEMA-to-glove contact is made. It may prove necessary to reapply the agent after six months if symptoms of sensitivity recur.

• Control of exacerbating occlusal factors – in some cases the loss of tooth substance is further exacerbated by a tooth-grinding habit. This may be controlled by affording disclusion of the teeth at times when grinding is thought to happen. The provision of a stabilisation splint can achieve this.

A stabilisation splint (Fig 4-7) is formed in the laboratory from hard acrylic. When worn by the patient, it

• discludes the teeth
• increases the occlusal vertical dimension (OVD)
• contacts all teeth evenly in centric relation
• provides protrusive and excursive guidance
• has no non-working interferences.

In so doing, it prevents tooth–to–tooth contact and may also be used as a diagnostic aid where subsequent treatment is planned to increase the OVD.

- Adhesive replacement of tooth substance – the morphology of the erosive lesion, often bounded by enamel, lends itself well to an adhesive approach. Where lost palatal tooth tissue is to be replaced in the upper anterior sextant, consideration must be given to the available space for such restorations. Often, due to compensatory tooth movement inter incisal space is not available and needs to be created. Two approaches to this problem may be adopted. Either space can be created by the Dahl principle before the restorations are placed, or the planned anterior restorations may be placed high, discluding the posterior teeth and allowing them in time to re-establish the occlusion by compensatory tooth movement. The traditional approach is to create space first, but this can significantly add to treatment time and requires good patient compliance in wearing and tolerating the necessary appliance.

Creating space orthodontically – this may be achieved by the Dahl principle. The original Dahl appliance consisted of an upper removable cobalt

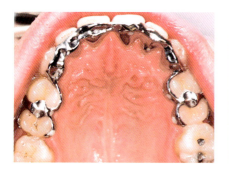

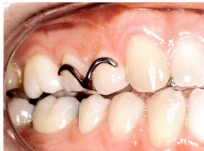

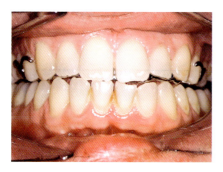

Fig 4-8 A Dahl appliance consisting of an upper removable cobalt chrome framework with 2mm coverage of the palatal aspects of the upper anterior teeth. Note the clasps engaging the buccal aspects of the canines and first premolars.

chrome framework with 2mm coverage of the palatal aspects of the upper anterior teeth. It was retained by clasps engaging the buccal aspects of the canines and first premolars (Fig 4-8). In a compliant patient it both intruded the lower incisors and enabled compensatory eruption of the posterior teeth. Thus, both the interincisal space and the morphological face height were increased (Fig 4-9). Upon removal, the need for posterior restorations - to maintain the increased face height - was eliminated due to posterior tooth to tooth contact achieved by compensatory eruption. In addition, the interincisal space created by the intrusion of the lower incisors permitted restoration. This appliance design may be adapted to address a wider variety of clinical situations including the presence of a diastema (Fig 4-10).

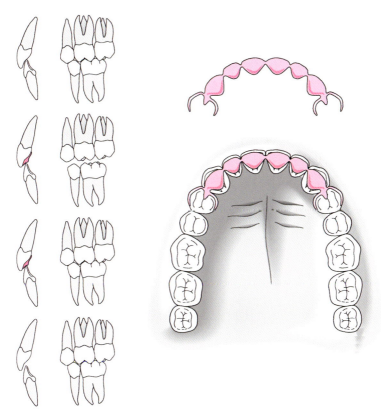

Fig 4-9 Diagrammatic illustration of how a Dahl appliance works to create interincisal space by enabling both lower incisor intrusion and compensatory eruption of molars.

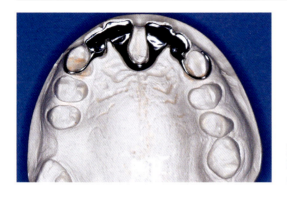

Fig 4-10 A modification of a Dahl appliance to take into account a mid-line diastema.

Sometimes, due to either a lack of retentive undercuts or poor patient compliance, the Dahl appliance may be cemented in place using a polycarboxylate or conventional glass polyalkenoate (ionomer) cement (Fig 4-11). Products that adhere to both tooth and metal should never be used as they will render the appliance near impossible to remove. Once space has been created, the appliance is removed. It is then essential that the palatal restorations are placed as soon as possible. A delay of just a week can result in loss of the interincisal space.

Creating space by restoration – the planned anterior restorations may be placed directly resulting in an apparently high restoration and disclusion of the posterior teeth. Generally, within two to three months the posterior occlusion re-establishes due to compensatory tooth eruption. An alternative strategy may be to provide, with no or, at most minimal tooth preparation, bilateral adhesively bonded gold or composite occlusal onlays upon selected posterior teeth (Fig 4-12). These should be placed in the same arch to sufficient height so as to open the bite anteriorly by 1-2mm. This creates the necessary interincisal clearance for palatal restoration of the maxillary anterior teeth. It also permits the posterior teeth to re-establish occlusion by compensatory tooth eruption. Such an approach is particularly useful when treating cases with both occlusal and palatal erosion. For optimum success the surface treatment of the onlay is of importance (see later in this chapter).

Occlusal infills and onlays – sometimes patients present with small eroded lesions on the occlusal aspect of posterior teeth. These are often acutely sensitive. Although the simplest way to restore such occlusal pits is by directly placed resin composite restorations these can sometimes repeatedly fail. A more predictable restoration is to place an adhesively bonded indirect resin composite restoration constructed in a laboratory from a silicone impression

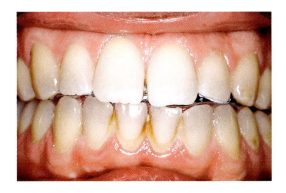

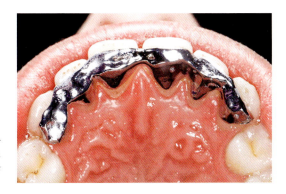

Fig 4-11 A fixed Dahl appliance temporarily cemented in place with polycarboxylate cement.

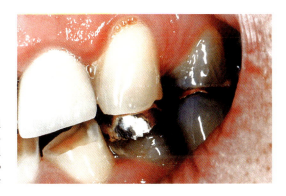

Fig 4-12 Adhesively bonded gold onlays LR4 and LR5 used to increase the occlusal vertical dimension in order to increase interincisal clearance

(Fig 4-13). Such composite has better physical properties with the greater degree of cross linking of the polymeric matrix afforded by the laboratory process of manufacture. Given the small size of these restorations, it is help-

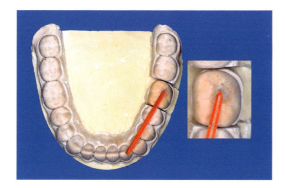

Fig 4-13 Indirect composite infill for an acutely sensitive occlusal pit. Note the handling spur that is removed using conventional high-speed rotary cutting instruments following cementation of the restoration.

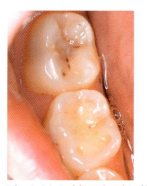 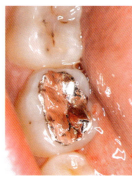 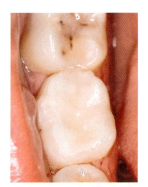

Fig 4-14 Gold occlusal infills contrasted with indirect resin composite infills made for the same patient.

ful to ask the laboratory to incorporate a spur of material upon the restoration. This assists in handling and orientation and is readily removed, with a conventional high speed rotary cutting instrument, once the restoration is bonded in place. Bonding may be achieved using a dual-cured resin composite luting system.

More extensive occlusal erosion, in sites subject to heavy occlusal loading, or where the surface is to be onlayed to increase the OVD, may be more durably restored with gold bonded to the residual tooth structure (Fig 4-14). This may however not be aesthetically acceptable to all patients so an indirect resin composite alternative may be required (see also Fig 4-14). Clearly, this needs to be discussed with the patient beforehand, as the appearance of bonded gold restorations may not match the aesthetic expectations of the patient. On the other hand gold demonstrates better wear resistance and exhibits greater

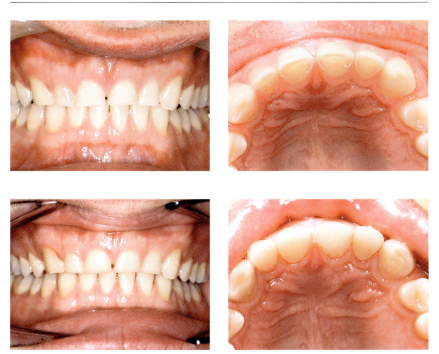

Fig 4-15 Indirect resin composite palatal veneers used to restore the palatal aspects of UR21 and UL12. Note the minimal impact upon the labial appearance of the teeth following restoration.

strength in thin section than resin composite. A chemically cured resin such as Panavia (Kuraray) should be used to bond the restoration in place. The gold alloy should be Type IV. To give optimum adhesion, the fitting surface should be grit-blasted with 50 micron lumina prior to cementation. Some would also suggest that oxidation of the restoration by the laboratory prior to cementation would further enhance bonding. If oxidation is to be carried out, it is essential that the alloy has a copper content of approximately 20%. It is this constituent that oxidises when the restoration is returned to the furnace to be held at 400°C for nine minutes prior to final placement.

Palatal and labial veneers – these restorations are relatively conservative of residual tooth structure. Indeed the tooth has often been prepared by the erosive process itself.

Palatal veneers – these may be placed where the enamel has been breached by the erosive process. Under such circumstances, the patient may be expe-

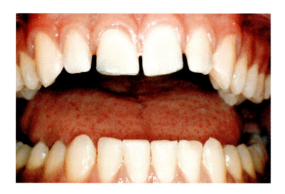

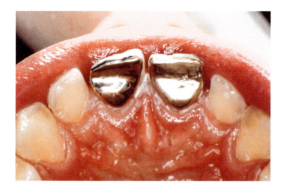

Fig 4-16 Gold palatal veneers UR1 and UL1 – note the bluish tinge to the incisal edges.

riencing dentine hypersensitivity and could be aware of a change in appearance in the labial aspect of the affected teeth. This may manifest as an alteration of the optical properties of the labial surface, or chipping of the incisal edge. An assessment of the available space for these restorations should be made. Study models, together with a diagnostic wax up, are useful to both determine this and to discuss with the patient any changes in tooth morphology, such as replacing lost incisal tooth tissue. This should include how the necessary space for the palatal veneers is to be created, and the type of material to be used in its construction.

The palatal veneer may be made of either resin composite or a Type IV gold alloy. Resin composite is tooth coloured and has relatively little impact on the labial appearance of the tooth (Fig 4-15). It is, however, a brittle material and prone to fracture in thin section. Upon partial fracture, it can either be repaired using dentine-bonded composite or the fractured edges simply

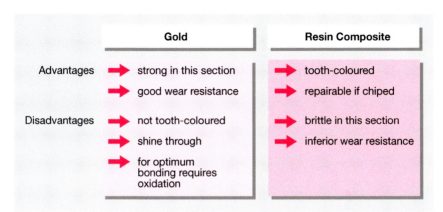

Fig 4-17 Some advantages and disadvantages of gold versus resin composite palatal veneers.

polished down for patient comfort. Gold is strong in thin sections and less abrasive to the opposing dentition. Its metallic appearance may give an unacceptable bluish tinge to the labial appearance and it does not lend itself to the aesthetic restoration of incisal edges that modern society demands (Fig 4-16). Both materials are adhesively bonded to the tooth using a combination of the acid etch technique and chemically active resins. For gold palatal veneers the gold alloy should be Type IV and to give optimum adhesion its fitting surface should be at least grit blasted with 50μm lumina prior to cementation with a chemically cured resin such as Panavia. Some would also suggest that oxidation of the restoration by the laboratory prior to cementation would further enhance bonding as previously described. Fig 4-17 summarises the merits and disadvantages of platal veneers made from gold or resin composite.

As such restorations will impact upon the appearance of the patient it is helpful to try in the restorations before cementation to both check their integrity and appearance. Due to their small size this can be problematical. The application of a small quantity of uncured visible light cured resin composite to the veneer prior to seating upon the tooth can be helpful. This is usually sufficiently sticky to allow the patient and dentist to assess the appearance and thereafter retrieve the restoration without difficulty. It can also be helpful to invite the patient to bring a close friend or relative along with them so that a second view can be obtained upon the aesthetic impact of the restoration.

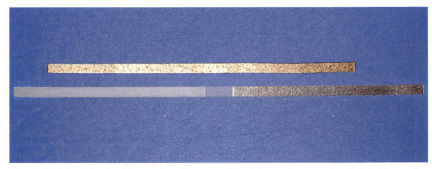

Fig 4-18 Metal backed (upper) and conventional (lower) approximal finishing strips – the former should be used with care so as not to lacerate the gingivae.

Once final cementation has been achieved, for optimum oral approximal oral hygiene, it is essential to ensure that no excess cement occludes the approximal spaces. Although this can usually be minimised by scrupulous removal prior to curing the cement it is occasionally necessary to use either conventional, or in extremis metal backed, approximal finishing strips (Fig 4-18). The patient must be instructed in the use of cleaning aids, such as dental floss, to maintain this area free from plaque.

In handling such restorations some may find the use of disposable self adhesive handling sticks of help (Fig 4-19). A variety of these exist and choice depends on the operator's personal preference. Some are stickier than others, and whereas this can be helpful it can also be a hindrance in releasing the restoration upon the tooths surface.

Labial veneers – where labial enamel has been affected by the erosive process consideration should be given to these restorations. They may either be provided as directly placed resin composite or in the form of indirect composite or porcelain veneers. If chipping of the veneers incisal edges are to be avoided, it is essential that an occlusal analysis is undertaken before the provision of such restorations. Any parafunctional activity likely to affect the integrity of the incisal edge, such as bruxism, should be ascertained before a decision is reached to provide the labial veneer. The appearance of a veneer restoration should be thoroughly scrutinised by the patient at try in before it is cemented. The presence of either a relative or close friend of the patient in the surgery can be of great assistance in this regard. Time should be taken

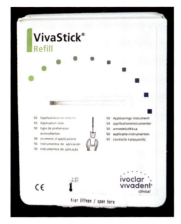

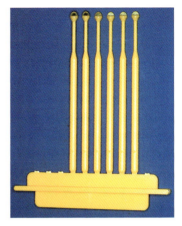

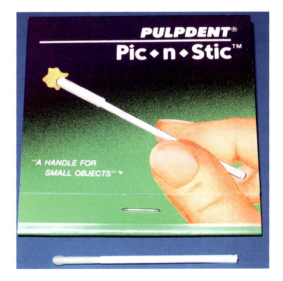

Fig 4-19 Examples of disposable self-adhesive handling sticks for use in manipulating small restorations.

to experiment and observe the effects upon appearance, of the use differing shades of veneer trial paste, before the final shade of veneer cement is selected (Fig 4-20).

Double veneers and dentine-bonded crowns – where both the labial and palatal surfaces have been affected, consideration may be given to the provision of these restorations.

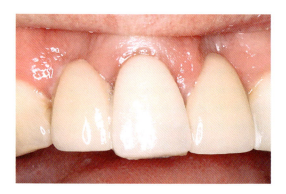

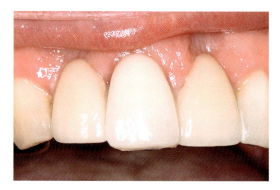

Fig 4-20 The effect of two different trial pastes upon the labial appearance of the labial veneer UR1.

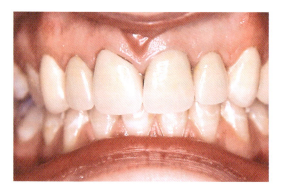

Fig 4-21 Dentine-bonded crowns upon the upper incisor teeth.

Dentine-bonded crowns (Fig 4-21) require often only minimal tooth preparation to eliminate mesial and distal undercuts and provide a distinct finishing line and space for the technician to produce an aesthetic labial

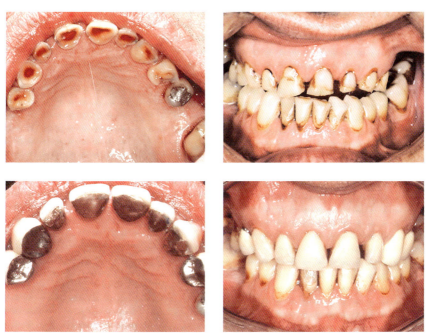

Fig 4-22 Case of severe palatal and labial tooth surface loss treated with double veneers – aetiology: excessive alcohol intake.

appearance that does not impact adversely from the emergence angle of the tooth. Theoretically they involve a reduced number of patient visits compared to double veneers. Great care must, however, be exercised in the choice of porcelain if fractures of the restoration are not to occur in function.

Double veneers (Fig 4-22) require relatively minimal tooth preparation. When combined with an increased OVD, stabilised with posterior restorations such as either crowns or adhesive gold onlays, they offer scope to address reduced incisal length as well as loss/discolouration of tooth substance. In such an application it is essential to protect the incisal edge of the labial veneer. This can be achieved by initially providing the palatal gold veneer to the increased incisal length and once it is cemented in place, preparing the labial surface for a porcelain veneer (Fig 4-23). Clearly at this stage a further impression is recorded so that the laboratory may make the labial veneer. A disadvantage is the rather unsightly appearance the patient

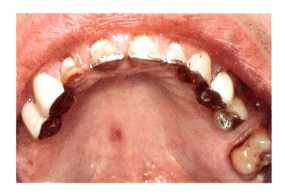

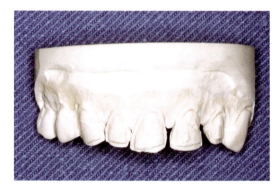

Fig 4-23 Gold palatal veneers cemented in place with labial preparation of the upper anteriors undertaken to accommodate an increased incisal length (same case as depicted in Figure 4-18).

is left with whilst awaiting the production of the labial veneer. As exposed structure remains in the approximal areas, following the cementation of both labial and palatal veneers, optimum approximal oral hygiene must be maintained by the patient.

Irrespective of the method of restoration once treatment is complete study casts should be obtained for use in future monitoring. It may be helpful to issue these to the patient so they have ownership of their future care.

Further Reading

Bishop K, Bell M, Briggs P, Kelleher M (1996) Restoration of a worn dentition using a double-veneer technique. British Dental Journal 1996;180:26-29.

Burke FJ. Treatment of loss of tooth substance using dentine-bonded crowns: report of a case. Dental Update 1998;25:235-240.

Chadwick RG, Linklater KI. A retrospective observational study of the effect of surface treatments and cementing media upon the durability of gold palatal veneers. Operative Dentistry 2004;29:608-613.

Dahl BL, Krogstad O. Long-term observations of an increased occlusal face height obtained by a combined orthodontic/prosthetic approach. Journal of Oral Rehabilitation 1985;12:173-176.

Redman CDJ, Hemmings K, Good JA. The survival and clinical performance of resin-based composite restorations used to treat localised anterior tooth wear. British Dental Journal 2003;194:566-572.

May J, Waterhouse PJ. Dental erosion and soft drinks: a qualitative assessment of knowledge, attitude and behaviour using focus groups of schoolchildren. A preliminary study. International Journal of Paediatric Dentistry 2003;13:425-433.

Chapter 5
The Future

Aim

To be appraised of emerging developments in the early diagnosis, monitoring, risk factor identification and prevention of dental erosion.

Outcome

After reading this chapter the practitioner should have an understanding of:
- Emerging technologies of potential assistance in making an early diagnosis of dental erosion.
- Potential future risk factor identification tools
- New potential preventive regimes.

The Future

Once a diagnosis of dental erosion has been made practitioners face a number of choices. They may elect to institute a preventive regime, with monitoring of tooth surface loss, or to intervene operatively. A balance has to be struck between the risks of further tooth substance loss occurring, should prevention fail, and providing restorative treatment that inevitably will require maintenance and replacement. Should the wrong decision be made the patient will either be condemned to unnecessary restorative treatment or future restorative options will be denied them due to a lack of tooth structure. Fig 5-1 illustrates such a dilemma. Are there any developments that may assist the dentist and the patient, either emerging now or likely to do so in the future? Especially in relation to early diagnosis and monitoring, identification of risk factors and new preventive regimes.

Early Diagnosis and Monitoring

Dental erosion arises from the loss of enamel and dentine from acid attack. It is therefore a consequence of the chemical process of demineralisation where gradual and sustained acid exposure progressively depletes the mineral content of the tooth. This ultimately culminates in a change in surface

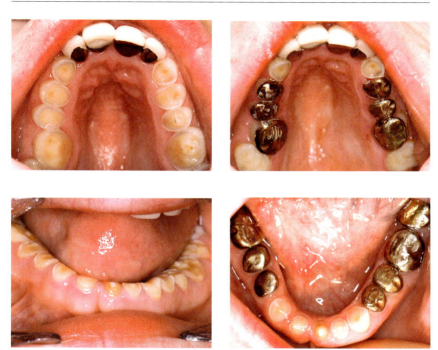

Fig 5-1 The dilemma of observing versus treatment – this extreme example illustrates how prolonged loss of tooth substance and zealous monitoring compromised tooth structure. Residual tooth structure was eventually protected by the provision of adhesively bonded gold onlays with no prior tooth preparation.

morphology. Much of this alteration in level of mineralisation occurs beneath the visible tooth surface. Eroded lesions are principally comprised of two distinct zones. The first is the defect formed by the actual loss of tooth substance. Beneath this is a layer of softened demineralised enamel/dentine that, given sufficient time and erosive challenge will be lost, contributing to further defect formation and a new softened tooth surface. It is relatively late in the erosive process when the tooth surface becomes changed in shape as surface softening must precede defect formation. Currently it is only then that the erosive process is highlighted to the dentist. If the early loss of mineral could in some way be detected before an alteration in surface morphology occurs preventive strategies could be put into place, that if successful, would conserve valuable tooth substance. No chairside technique currently exists to assess changes in mineral content, although in the laboratory quantitative light-induced fluoresence (QLF) has successfully been used to quan-

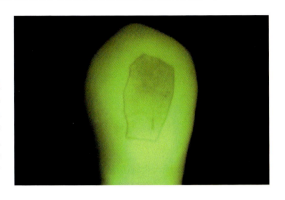

Fig 5-2 Laboratory generated erosion of human tooth as viewed using QLF. The area that is unaffected is the windowed area. This buccal area was protected from the erosive attack of orange juice by a coating of nail varnish.

tify mineral loss. In essence, sound coronal tooth substance, when subjected to a beam of monochromatic blue light of a wavelength of 370nm, fluoresces yellow-green. This can be measured and compared to eroded tissue where the scattering of the light, due to increased porosity, reduces the level of auto-fluoresence (Fig 5-2). Much development work however, still needs to be carried out on this useful laboratory tool if it is to develop into a chairside test.

Currently it is universally recognised that study models, recorded at sequential intervals, are useful for monitoring the progression of tooth surface loss and assessing the impact of preventive advice upon the erosive process. They are however, both bulky and fragile. Although valuable storage space may be saved in the surgery by issuing them to the patient for safe keeping they could well become lost or broken resulting in the loss of much valuable information. The use of digital study model capture and storage systems, although potentially rendering conventional study models obsolete in the future, is still in its infancy. Despite this the detection capacity of ongoing tooth surface loss, by comparing sequential study casts, is relatively gross and insufficiently sensitive to assess the subtle early impact of preventive measures – such as an alteration in dietary intake. This therefore misses an important opportunity to educate and motivate patients by illustrating to them that their change in lifestyle has slowed or ceased the rate of tooth surface loss. Within the research community, in recent years, there has been some use of surface mapping techniques to quantify the degree of tooth surface loss. Such measurement is made difficult by the lack of fixed reference points within the oral cavity as required by all conventional measurement techniques. As a consequence surface matching and difference detection techniques have been developed. These are used to compare digital terrain models (DTM's)

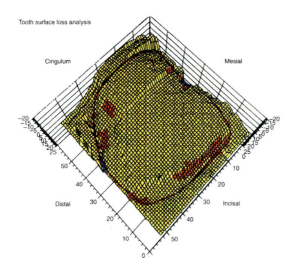

Tooth surface loss analysis

Cingulum

Mesial

Distal

Incisal

Fig 5-3 A colour-coded surface difference plot of the palatal aspect of a maxillary central incisor following palatal surface loss. The site of wear is shown together with the degree of loss as represented by colour-coding.

of the teeth, recorded at different intervals of time. The changes in tooth morphology are shown as colour coded surface plots (Fig 5-3) that indicate both the site and magnitude of surface loss. Although such techniques have been applied in epidemiological investigations they are very labour intensive and as yet are not sufficiently developed for chairside application.

Epidemiological surveys of tooth surface loss generally utilise descriptive indices to categorize the severity of tooth surface loss. Although a number have been developed over the years they have not achieved anything like universal acceptance and certainly are not used by dentists to assess the rate of ongoing tooth surface loss. This is because they are complex, difficult to learn and time consuming to apply. Some score the dentition directly, usually involving some assessment of the extent of exposed dentine, whereas others involve a detailed examination of sequential study casts. If one reflects upon the advances in screening and coding for periodontal disease using the Basic Periodontal Examination (BPE), that have occurred over the last decade, in dental practice it is likely and desirable that a universally recognised index for monitoring tooth surface loss will be developed. This would be an important tool for the busy practitioner.

Identification of Risk Factors

It is now apparent that although the presence of either extrinsic or intrinsic acid is a pre requisite for dental erosion to develop it is not a simple cause and effect relationship. Individual susceptibility plays a major role. The precise mechanisms are poorly understood. Although potential risk factors have been discussed earlier in this book (See Chapter 2) emerging developments in the areas of salivary assays and better liaison with the general medical practitioner warrant further comment.

Developments in salivary assays – As well as the obvious clearance and buffering functions saliva, by the action of some of its protein components (acidic proline-rich proteins, histatins and cystatins), inhibits the precipitation of calcium and phosphate salts. Although currently salivary flow rate and buffer capacity may be assayed by commercially available test kits no chairside test may assay the inhibitory effects of these protein components. Although it is as yet unclear as to the significance of such activity for dental erosion saliva's inhibition of the precipitation of calcium and phosphate salts in the oral cavity is receiving some attention in the research community. Inhibition of the precipitation of calcium phosphates is crucial in maintaining the mineral structure of enamel which is in continuous contact with the saliva. This body fluid is itself supersaturated with respect to calcium phosphate salts. At the same time precipitation of such salts is necessary to promote remineralisation of tooth substance. Clearly an equilibrium exists between the two requirements. This could be upset against remineralisation according to the mix of protein variants present in the saliva. Potentially this could favour the development of dental erosion and account in part for an individuals susceptibility to erosion. The outcome of research to prove or disprove this hypothesis is awaited for, if proven, a susceptibility test may result.

Better general medical practitioner liaison – It has been shown that those patients who either complain of symptoms of gastro oesophageal disease (GORD) and those diagnosed with this condition have a greater prevalence of tooth wear involving dentine. Estimates of the prevalence of GORD range from 6-10%. By observing dental erosion early, and referring through the general medical practitioner for further investigation of its aetiology, the dentist may play a pivotal role in the early diagnosis of this medical condition. Although such referral protocols are the norm in some geographic areas this is not the case in all. A greater awareness of the link by both the medical and dental professions would clearly help in the management of such patients. Undiagnosed and untreated GORD may result in oesophagitis, Barrett's epithelium, oesophageal adenocarcinoma and aspirational pneumonitis of various degrees (Fig 5-4). Its clinical presentation includes heartburn, non cardiac chest pain, chronic cough and hoarseness together with gastric juice in the mouth, chronic sore throat and laryngeal carcinoma. There is as yet

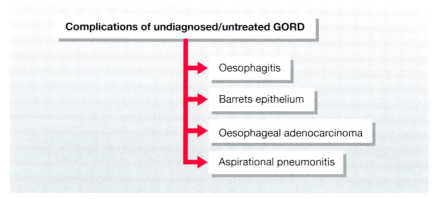

Fig 5-4 Complications of undiagnosed/untreated GORD.

no single test that can consistently detect GORD. Currently the most useful diagnostic tool available is 24 hour monitoring of the oesophageal pH. A pH, in the distal oesophagus, less than 4.0 for 4% of the time is considered pathological. Treatment may be by means of either non pharmacological or pharmacological methods. Non–pharmacological methods include the simple elevation of the bed head and the avoidance of fatty and spicy foods. Histamine – 2 (H2) blockers or proton–pump inhibitors may be prescribed as well as drugs that enhance gastric motility. Surgical intervention (Nissen fundoplication) may be necessary when these measures fail.

New Preventive Regimes

It is interesting to note that the drinks manufacturers seem aware of the potential dangers for the dentition of consuming excessive quantities of acidic drinks. It is an unfortunate fact that acid is necessary in many beverages and foods to give both flavour and taste perception. Product stability is also enhanced by its presence. These properties contribute to the market share a product has. Notwithstanding this, and perhaps driven by market considerations, some manufacturers have sought to promote low acid content variants with some impact upon the titratable acidity of the drink (Table 5-1). Other means of reducing the erosive effects of drinks have included both increasing the quantities of ionised calcium and phosphate within the drink or adding fluoride to it. These approaches are however not without their own problems. Although increased quantities of calcium and phosphate will suppress demineralisation of tooth substance by lessening the movement of these ions out of the tooth, upon exposure to the drink, by the law of mass

Table 5-1 The effect of commercially available product modification upon the pH and titratable acidity of a fresh orange juice.

	Tropicana Pure Premium Orange	Tropicana Essentials – Orange Low Acid	Tropicana Essentials – Orange with Calcium
Mean pH	3.44 (0.46)	3.89 (0.06)	3.93 (0.01)
Mean titratable acidity	24.76 (1.24)	19.10 (0.98)	22.02 (1.06)

★Note the statistically significant increase in pH ($P < 0.05$) and reduction in titratable acidity ($P < 0.01$) that these product modifications confer.

★Means derived from five samples of 25ml of each drink. Titratable acidity is the volume of 0.1 molar sodium hydroxide required to raise the pH to 7.0. Parenthesised values are the standard deviations of the observations.

action their presence impairs flavour. This may necessitate the addition of more acid, thus obviating the beneficial effect. Although fluoride could be added to facilitate remineralisation an insurmountable problem then arises for it is impossible to safely control the fluoride dosage that each consumer will receive. Ultimately however, it is the consumer who dictates what level of product modification is acceptable for if found to be unpalatable the product will not be bought again. There is thus also the risk of brand tarnishing so to offer such alternatives in a product range is not without considerable financial risk.

In Chapter 4 the potential of a new commercial product to control further tooth substance loss, based upon the milk protein CPP – ACP (casein phosphopeptide – amorphous calcium phosphate), was discussed. Its efficacy in this regard is as yet unclear.

Another approach, currently under investigation, to protect the worn palatal surfaces of teeth from further acid attack is the application of wet dentine-bonding resins to such surfaces. This potentially substitutes the protective effects that the salivary pellicle confers against erosion in situations where, due to active and aggressive erosion, a pellicle may not be present to sufficient extent to offer protection. Such a protective coating may lack sufficient wear resistance so an alternative may be to use resin fissure sealants bonded to the dentine by the application of a suitable dentine bonding agent. The results of clinical trials of such innovative approaches are awaited with interest.

Postscript

Reflecting back on the quotation of G. V. Black that began this book, it is interesting to note that, despite much research activity in the intervening 100 years, our information regarding erosion is still far from complete.

Further Reading

Barron RP, Carmichael RP, Marcon MA. Sandor GKB. Dental erosion in gastroesophageal reflux disease. Journal of the Canadian Dental Association 2003;69:84–89.

Chadwick RG, Mitchell HL. Presentation of quantitative tooth wear data to clinicians. Quintessence International 1999;30:393–398.

Hooper SM, Meredith N, Jagger DC. The development of a new index for measurement of incisal/occlusal tooth wear. Journal of Oral Rehabilitation 2004;31:206-212.

Mitchell HL, Chadwick RG. Mathematical shape matching as a tool in tooth wear assessment – development and conduct. Journal of Oral Rehabilitation 1998;25:921-928.

Pretty IA, Edgar WM. Higham SM. The erosive potential of commercially available mouthrinses on enamel as measured by Quantitative Light-induced Fluorescence (QLF). Journal of Dentistry 2003;31:313-319.

Sundaram G, Bartlett D, Watson T. Bonding to and protecting worn palatal surfaces of teeth with dentine bonding agents. Journal of Oral Rehabilitation 2004;31:505-509.

Index

Quintessentials for General Dental Practitioners Series

in 50 volumes

Editor-in-Chief: Professor Nairn H F Wilson

General Dentistry, Editor: Nairn Wilson

Implantology in General Dental Practice	available
Culturally Sensitive Oral Healthcare	available
Dental Erosion	available
Managing Orofacial Pain in Practice	Autumn 2006
Dental Bleaching	Autumn 2006
Special Care Dentistry	Autumn 2006
Infection Control for the Dental Team	Spring 2007
Therapeutics and Medical Emergencies in the Everyday Clinical Practice of Dentistry	Spring 2007

Oral Surgery and Oral Medicine, Editor: John G Meechan

Practical Dental Local Anaesthesia	available
Practical Oral Medicine	available
Practical Conscious Sedation	available
Minor Oral Surgery in Dental Practice	available

Imaging, Editor: Keith Horner

Interpreting Dental Radiographs	available
Panoramic Radiology	available
Twenty-first Century Dental Imaging	Autumn 2006

Periodontology, Editor: Iain L C Chapple

Understanding Periodontal Diseases: Assessment and Diagnostic Procedures in Practice	available
Decision-Making for the Periodontal Team	available
Successful Periodontal Therapy – A Non-Surgical Approach	available
Periodontal Management of Children, Adolescents and Young Adults	available
Periodontal Medicine: A Window on the Body	available

Endodontics, Editor: John M Whitworth

Rational Root Canal Treatment in Practice	available
Managing Endodontic Failure in Practice	available
Restoring Endodontically Treated Teeth	Autumn 2006

Prosthodontics, Editor: P Finbarr Allen

Teeth for Life for Older Adults	available
Complete Dentures – from Planning to Problem Solving	available
Removable Partial Dentures	available
Fixed Prosthodontics in Dental Practice	available
Occlusion: A Theoretical and Team Approach	Autumn 2006

Operative Dentistry, Editor: Paul A Brunton

Decision-Making in Operative Dentistry	available
Aesthetic Dentistry	available
Communicating in Dental Practice	available
Indirect Restorations	Summer 2006
Choosing and Using Dental Materials	Autumn 2006

Paediatric Dentistry/Orthodontics, Editor: Marie Therese Hosey

Child Taming: How to Cope with Children in Dental Practice	available
Paediatric Cariology	available
Treatment Planning for the Developing Dentition	available
Managing Dental Trauma in Practice	available

General Dentistry and Practice Management, Editor: Raj Rattan

The Business of Dentistry	available
Risk Management	available
Quality Matters: From Clinical Care to Customer Service	Summer 2006
Practice Management for the Dental Team	Autumn 2006
Dental Practice Design	Autumn 2006
Handling Complaint in Dental Practice	Autumn 2006

Dental Team, Editor: Mabel Slater

Team Players in Dentistry	Autumn 2006

Quintessence Publishing Co. Ltd., London